Today's Goal _______________ (M) (T) (W) (T) (F) ●S ●S

Muscle Group Focus _______________   Weight ________   Date/Time __________

Stretch ◯   Warm-Up _________________________________

Strength Training

Exercise		Set 1	Set 2	Set 3	Set 4	Set 5	Set 6
	Reps						
	Weight						
	Reps						
	Weight						
	Reps						
	Weight						
	Reps						
	Weight						
	Reps						
	Weight						
	Reps						
	Weight						
	Reps						
	Weight						
	Reps						
	Weight						
	Reps						
	Weight						

Cardio

Exercise	Calories	Distance	Time

Water Intake _________________

Cooldown _________________

Feeling ☆ ☆ ☆ ☆ ☆

Notes

Today's Goal ____________   M T W T F S S

Muscle Group Focus ____________   Weight ________   Date/Time ________

Stretch ○   Warm-Up ____________

Strength Training

Exercise		Set 1	Set 2	Set 3	Set 4	Set 5	Set 6
	Reps						
	Weight						
	Reps						
	Weight						
	Reps						
	Weight						
	Reps						
	Weight						
	Reps						
	Weight						
	Reps						
	Weight						
	Reps						
	Weight						
	Reps						
	Weight						
	Reps						
	Weight						

Cardio

Exercise	Calories	Distance	Time

Water Intake ____________

Cooldown ____________

Feeling ☆ ☆ ☆ ☆ ☆

Notes

Today's Goal _______________   Ⓜ Ⓣ Ⓦ Ⓣ Ⓕ Ⓢ Ⓢ

Muscle Group Focus _______________   Weight _______   Date/Time _______

Stretch ◯   Warm-Up _______________

Strength Training

Exercise		Set 1	Set 2	Set 3	Set 4	Set 5	Set 6
	Reps						
	Weight						
	Reps						
	Weight						
	Reps						
	Weight						
	Reps						
	Weight						
	Reps						
	Weight						
	Reps						
	Weight						
	Reps						
	Weight						
	Reps						
	Weight						
	Reps						
	Weight						

Cardio

Exercise	Calories	Distance	Time

Water Intake _______________

Cooldown _______________

Feeling ☆ ☆ ☆ ☆ ☆

Notes

Today's Goal ___________________ Ⓜ Ⓣ Ⓦ Ⓣ Ⓕ ⬤S ⬤S

Muscle Group Focus ______________   Weight ________   Date/Time _________

Stretch ◯   Warm-Up ____

Strength Training

Exercise		Set 1	Set 2	Set 3	Set 4	Set 5	Set 6
	Reps						
	Weight						
	Reps						
	Weight						
	Reps						
	Weight						
	Reps						
	Weight						
	Reps						
	Weight						
	Reps						
	Weight						
	Reps						
	Weight						
	Reps						
	Weight						
	Reps						
	Weight						

Cardio

Exercise	Calories	Distance	Time

Water Intake _______________

Cooldown _______________

Feeling ☆ ☆ ☆ ☆ ☆

Notes

Today's Goal

Today's Goal ______________ M T W T F **S** **S**

Muscle Group Focus ______________   Weight ________   Date/Time ______________

Stretch ◯   Warm-Up ______________________________________

Strength Training

Exercise		Set 1	Set 2	Set 3	Set 4	Set 5	Set 6
	Reps						
	Weight						
	Reps						
	Weight						
	Reps						
	Weight						
	Reps						
	Weight						
	Reps						
	Weight						
	Reps						
	Weight						
	Reps						
	Weight						
	Reps						
	Weight						
	Reps						
	Weight						

Cardio

Exercise	Calories	Distance	Time

Water Intake ______________

Cooldown ______________

Feeling ☆ ☆ ☆ ☆ ☆

Notes

Today's Goal ________________   (M) (T) (W) (T) (F) (S) (S)

Muscle Group Focus ________________   Weight ________   Date/Time ________

Stretch ◯   Warm-Up ________________

Strength Training

Exercise		Set 1	Set 2	Set 3	Set 4	Set 5	Set 6
	Reps						
	Weight						
	Reps						
	Weight						
	Reps						
	Weight						
	Reps						
	Weight						
	Reps						
	Weight						
	Reps						
	Weight						
	Reps						
	Weight						
	Reps						
	Weight						
	Reps						
	Weight						
	Reps						
	Weight						

Cardio

Exercise	Calories	Distance	Time

Water Intake ________________

Cooldown ________________

Feeling ☆ ☆ ☆ ☆ ☆

Notes

Today's Goal   __________   (M) (T) (W) (T) (F) (S) (S)

Muscle Group Focus __________   Weight ________   Date/Time __________

Stretch ◯   Warm-Up __________________________________

Strength Training

Exercise		Set 1	Set 2	Set 3	Set 4	Set 5	Set 6
	Reps						
	Weight						
	Reps						
	Weight						
	Reps						
	Weight						
	Reps						
	Weight						
	Reps						
	Weight						
	Reps						
	Weight						
	Reps						
	Weight						
	Reps						
	Weight						
	Reps						
	Weight						
	Reps						
	Weight						

Cardio

Exercise	Calories	Distance	Time

Water Intake __________________

Cooldown __________________

Feeling ☆ ☆ ☆ ☆ ☆

Notes

Today's Goal

(M) (T) (W) (T) (F) (**S**) (**S**)

Muscle Group Focus ___________________   Weight _________   Date/Time _________

Stretch ◯   Warm-Up ___________________________________

Strength Training

Exercise		Set 1	Set 2	Set 3	Set 4	Set 5	Set 6
	Reps						
	Weight						
	Reps						
	Weight						
	Reps						
	Weight						
	Reps						
	Weight						
	Reps						
	Weight						
	Reps						
	Weight						
	Reps						
	Weight						
	Reps						
	Weight						
	Reps						
	Weight						
	Reps						
	Weight						

Cardio

Exercise	Calories	Distance	Time

Water Intake ___________________

Cooldown ___________________

Feeling ☆ ☆ ☆ ☆ ☆

Notes

Today's Goal _______________   Ⓜ Ⓣ Ⓦ Ⓣ Ⓕ Ⓢ Ⓢ

Muscle Group Focus _______________   Weight _______   Date/Time _______

Stretch ◯   Warm-Up _______________________________

Strength Training

Exercise		Set 1	Set 2	Set 3	Set 4	Set 5	Set 6
	Reps						
	Weight						
	Reps						
	Weight						
	Reps						
	Weight						
	Reps						
	Weight						
	Reps						
	Weight						
	Reps						
	Weight						
	Reps						
	Weight						
	Reps						
	Weight						
	Reps						
	Weight						

Cardio

Exercise	Calories	Distance	Time

Water Intake _______________

Cooldown _______________

Feeling ☆ ☆ ☆ ☆ ☆

Notes

Today's Goal ________________   Ⓜ Ⓣ Ⓦ Ⓣ Ⓕ ⬤ ⬤

Muscle Group Focus ________________   Weight ________   Date/Time ________

Stretch ◯   Warm-Up ________________________________

Strength Training

Exercise		Set 1	Set 2	Set 3	Set 4	Set 5	Set 6
	Reps						
	Weight						
	Reps						
	Weight						
	Reps						
	Weight						
	Reps						
	Weight						
	Reps						
	Weight						
	Reps						
	Weight						
	Reps						
	Weight						
	Reps						
	Weight						
	Reps						
	Weight						
	Reps						
	Weight						

Cardio

Exercise	Calories	Distance	Time

Water Intake ________________

Cooldown ________________

Feeling ☆ ☆ ☆ ☆ ☆

Notes

Today's Goal ______________ Ⓜ Ⓣ Ⓦ Ⓣ Ⓕ **Ⓢ** **Ⓢ**

Muscle Group Focus ______________   Weight ________   Date/Time __________

Stretch ◯   Warm-Up ___________________________________

Strength Training

Exercise		Set 1	Set 2	Set 3	Set 4	Set 5	Set 6
	Reps						
	Weight						
	Reps						
	Weight						
	Reps						
	Weight						
	Reps						
	Weight						
	Reps						
	Weight						
	Reps						
	Weight						
	Reps						
	Weight						
	Reps						
	Weight						
	Reps						
	Weight						

Cardio

Exercise	Calories	Distance	Time

Water Intake __________

Cooldown __________

Feeling ☆ ☆ ☆ ☆ ☆

Notes

Today's Goal ______________   (M) (T) (W) (T) (F) (S) (S)

Muscle Group Focus ______________   Weight ______   Date/Time ______

Stretch ◯   Warm-Up ______________

Strength Training

Exercise		Set 1	Set 2	Set 3	Set 4	Set 5	Set 6
	Reps						
	Weight						
	Reps						
	Weight						
	Reps						
	Weight						
	Reps						
	Weight						
	Reps						
	Weight						
	Reps						
	Weight						
	Reps						
	Weight						
	Reps						
	Weight						
	Reps						
	Weight						
	Reps						
	Weight						

Cardio

Exercise	Calories	Distance	Time

Water Intake ______________

Cooldown ______________

Feeling ☆ ☆ ☆ ☆ ☆

Notes

Today's Goal ___________ (M) (T) (W) (T) (F) **(S) (S)**

Muscle Group Focus ___________   Weight ________   Date/Time ___________

Stretch ◯   Warm-Up ___________________________________

Strength Training

Exercise		Set 1	Set 2	Set 3	Set 4	Set 5	Set 6
	Reps						
	Weight						
	Reps						
	Weight						
	Reps						
	Weight						
	Reps						
	Weight						
	Reps						
	Weight						
	Reps						
	Weight						
	Reps						
	Weight						
	Reps						
	Weight						
	Reps						
	Weight						
	Reps						
	Weight						

Cardio

Exercise	Calories	Distance	Time

Water Intake ___________

Cooldown ___________

Feeling ☆ ☆ ☆ ☆ ☆

Notes

Today's Goal ___________ (M) (T) (W) (T) (F) (S) (S)

Muscle Group Focus ___________ Weight _______ Date/Time _______

Stretch ○ Warm-Up _______________________

Strength Training

Exercise		Set 1	Set 2	Set 3	Set 4	Set 5	Set 6
	Reps						
	Weight						
	Reps						
	Weight						
	Reps						
	Weight						
	Reps						
	Weight						
	Reps						
	Weight						
	Reps						
	Weight						
	Reps						
	Weight						
	Reps						
	Weight						
	Reps						
	Weight						
	Reps						
	Weight						

Cardio

Exercise	Calories	Distance	Time

Water Intake _______________

Cooldown _______________

Feeling ☆ ☆ ☆ ☆ ☆

Notes

Today's Goal _______________   Ⓜ Ⓣ Ⓦ Ⓣ Ⓕ ⚫S ⚫S

Muscle Group Focus _______________   Weight _______   Date/Time _______

Stretch ◯   Warm-Up _______________________________

Strength Training

Exercise		Set 1	Set 2	Set 3	Set 4	Set 5	Set 6
	Reps						
	Weight						
	Reps						
	Weight						
	Reps						
	Weight						
	Reps						
	Weight						
	Reps						
	Weight						
	Reps						
	Weight						
	Reps						
	Weight						
	Reps						
	Weight						
	Reps						
	Weight						

Cardio

Exercise	Calories	Distance	Time

Water Intake _______________

Cooldown _______________

Feeling ☆ ☆ ☆ ☆ ☆

Notes

Today's Goal ____________________ (M) (T) (W) (T) (F) (S) (S)

Muscle Group Focus ____________   Weight ______   Date/Time __________

Stretch ◯   Warm-Up ______________________________________

Strength Training

Exercise		Set 1	Set 2	Set 3	Set 4	Set 5	Set 6
	Reps						
	Weight						
	Reps						
	Weight						
	Reps						
	Weight						
	Reps						
	Weight						
	Reps						
	Weight						
	Reps						
	Weight						
	Reps						
	Weight						
	Reps						
	Weight						
	Reps						
	Weight						
	Reps						
	Weight						

Cardio

Exercise	Calories	Distance	Time
______			
______			
______			

Water Intake ________________

Cooldown ________________

Feeling ☆ ☆ ☆ ☆ ☆

Notes

Today's Goal ___________ Ⓜ Ⓣ Ⓦ Ⓣ Ⓕ Ⓢ Ⓢ

Muscle Group Focus ___________ Weight ________ Date/Time ___________

Stretch ◯   Warm-Up ______________________________________

Strength Training

Exercise		Set 1	Set 2	Set 3	Set 4	Set 5	Set 6
	Reps						
	Weight						
	Reps						
	Weight						
	Reps						
	Weight						
	Reps						
	Weight						
	Reps						
	Weight						
	Reps						
	Weight						
	Reps						
	Weight						
	Reps						
	Weight						
	Reps						
	Weight						

Cardio

Exercise	Calories	Distance	Time

Water Intake ___________

Cooldown ___________

Feeling ☆ ☆ ☆ ☆ ☆

Notes

Today's Goal

<u>M</u> <u>T</u> <u>W</u> <u>T</u> <u>F</u> **S** **S**

Muscle Group Focus ______________   Weight ________   Date/Time __________

Stretch ◯   Warm-Up ________________________________

Strength Training

Exercise		Set 1	Set 2	Set 3	Set 4	Set 5	Set 6
	Reps						
	Weight						
	Reps						
	Weight						
	Reps						
	Weight						
	Reps						
	Weight						
	Reps						
	Weight						
	Reps						
	Weight						
	Reps						
	Weight						
	Reps						
	Weight						
	Reps						
	Weight						
	Reps						
	Weight						

Cardio

Exercise	Calories	Distance	Time

Water Intake ________________

Cooldown ________________

Feeling ☆ ☆ ☆ ☆ ☆

Notes

Today's Goal ___________   Ⓜ Ⓣ Ⓦ Ⓣ Ⓕ ⚫S ⚫S

Muscle Group Focus ___________   Weight _______   Date/Time ___________

Stretch ◯   Warm-Up ___________________________

Strength Training

Exercise		Set 1	Set 2	Set 3	Set 4	Set 5	Set 6
	Reps						
	Weight						
	Reps						
	Weight						
	Reps						
	Weight						
	Reps						
	Weight						
	Reps						
	Weight						
	Reps						
	Weight						
	Reps						
	Weight						
	Reps						
	Weight						
	Reps						
	Weight						
	Reps						
	Weight						

Cardio

Exercise	Calories	Distance	Time

Water Intake ___________

Cooldown ___________

Feeling ☆ ☆ ☆ ☆ ☆

Notes

Today's Goal ____________________ Ⓜ Ⓣ Ⓦ Ⓣ Ⓕ **S** **S**

Muscle Group Focus ____________________ Weight ________ Date/Time ________

Stretch ◯   Warm-Up ____________________

Strength Training

Exercise		Set 1	Set 2	Set 3	Set 4	Set 5	Set 6
	Reps						
	Weight						
	Reps						
	Weight						
	Reps						
	Weight						
	Reps						
	Weight						
	Reps						
	Weight						
	Reps						
	Weight						
	Reps						
	Weight						
	Reps						
	Weight						
	Reps						
	Weight						
	Reps						
	Weight						

Cardio

Exercise	Calories	Distance	Time

Water Intake ____________________

Cooldown ____________________

Feeling ☆ ☆ ☆ ☆ ☆

Notes

Today's Goal _______________   (M) (T) (W) (T) (F) (S) (S)

Muscle Group Focus _______________   Weight _______   Date/Time _______

Stretch ◯   Warm-Up _______________________________

Strength Training

Exercise		Set 1	Set 2	Set 3	Set 4	Set 5	Set 6
	Reps						
	Weight						
	Reps						
	Weight						
	Reps						
	Weight						
	Reps						
	Weight						
	Reps						
	Weight						
	Reps						
	Weight						
	Reps						
	Weight						
	Reps						
	Weight						
	Reps						
	Weight						

Cardio

Exercise	Calories	Distance	Time

Water Intake _______________

Cooldown _______________

Feeling ☆ ☆ ☆ ☆ ☆

Notes

Today's Goal _______________ Ⓜ Ⓣ Ⓦ Ⓣ Ⓕ ⬤S ⬤S

Muscle Group Focus _____________   Weight _______   Date/Time _______

Stretch ◯   Warm-Up _____________________________

Strength Training

Exercise		Set 1	Set 2	Set 3	Set 4	Set 5	Set 6
	Reps						
	Weight						
	Reps						
	Weight						
	Reps						
	Weight						
	Reps						
	Weight						
	Reps						
	Weight						
	Reps						
	Weight						
	Reps						
	Weight						
	Reps						
	Weight						
	Reps						
	Weight						

Cardio

Exercise	Calories	Distance	Time

Water Intake _____________

Cooldown _____________

Feeling ☆ ☆ ☆ ☆ ☆

Notes

Today's Goal ____________________ Ⓜ Ⓣ Ⓦ Ⓣ Ⓕ 🅢 🅢

Muscle Group Focus ________________   Weight ________   Date/Time __________

Stretch ◯   Warm-Up ____

Strength Training

Exercise		Set 1	Set 2	Set 3	Set 4	Set 5	Set 6
	Reps						
	Weight						
	Reps						
	Weight						
	Reps						
	Weight						
	Reps						
	Weight						
	Reps						
	Weight						
	Reps						
	Weight						
	Reps						
	Weight						
	Reps						
	Weight						
	Reps						
	Weight						

Cardio

Exercise	Calories	Distance	Time

Water Intake ___________________

Cooldown ___________________

Feeling ☆ ☆ ☆ ☆ ☆

Notes

Today's Goal ________________   (M) (T) (W) (T) (F) (S) (S)

Muscle Group Focus ________________   Weight ________   Date/Time ________

Stretch ◯   Warm-Up ________________

Strength Training

Exercise		Set 1	Set 2	Set 3	Set 4	Set 5	Set 6
	Reps						
	Weight						
	Reps						
	Weight						
	Reps						
	Weight						
	Reps						
	Weight						
	Reps						
	Weight						
	Reps						
	Weight						
	Reps						
	Weight						
	Reps						
	Weight						
	Reps						
	Weight						
	Reps						
	Weight						

Cardio

Exercise	Calories	Distance	Time

Water Intake ________________

Cooldown ________________

Feeling ☆ ☆ ☆ ☆ ☆

Notes

Today's Goal   _____________________   (M) (T) (W) (T) (F) (S) (S)

Muscle Group Focus _____________________   Weight ________   Date/Time ___________

Stretch ◯   Warm-Up _____________________________________

Strength Training

Exercise		Set 1	Set 2	Set 3	Set 4	Set 5	Set 6
	Reps						
	Weight						
	Reps						
	Weight						
	Reps						
	Weight						
	Reps						
	Weight						
	Reps						
	Weight						
	Reps						
	Weight						
	Reps						
	Weight						
	Reps						
	Weight						
	Reps						
	Weight						
	Reps						
	Weight						

Cardio

Exercise	Calories	Distance	Time

Water Intake _____________________

Cooldown _____________________

Feeling ☆ ☆ ☆ ☆ ☆

Notes

Today's Goal ___________________ (M) (T) (W) (T) (F) (S) (S)

Muscle Group Focus ___________________   Weight _______   Date/Time __________

Stretch ◯   Warm-Up ____________________________________

Strength Training

Exercise		Set 1	Set 2	Set 3	Set 4	Set 5	Set 6
	Reps						
	Weight						
	Reps						
	Weight						
	Reps						
	Weight						
	Reps						
	Weight						
	Reps						
	Weight						
	Reps						
	Weight						
	Reps						
	Weight						
	Reps						
	Weight						
	Reps						
	Weight						
	Reps						
	Weight						

Cardio

Exercise	Calories	Distance	Time

Water Intake ____________________

Cooldown ____________________

Feeling ☆ ☆ ☆ ☆ ☆

Notes

Today's Goal ___________________ (M) (T) (W) (T) (F) **(S)** **(S)**

Muscle Group Focus ___________ Weight _______ Date/Time __________

Stretch ○   Warm-Up ___________________________________

Strength Training

Exercise		Set 1	Set 2	Set 3	Set 4	Set 5	Set 6
	Reps						
	Weight						
	Reps						
	Weight						
	Reps						
	Weight						
	Reps						
	Weight						
	Reps						
	Weight						
	Reps						
	Weight						
	Reps						
	Weight						
	Reps						
	Weight						
	Reps						
	Weight						

Cardio

Exercise	Calories	Distance	Time

Water Intake ___________________

Cooldown ___________________

Feeling ☆ ☆ ☆ ☆ ☆

Notes

Today's Goal ____________   Ⓜ Ⓣ Ⓦ Ⓣ Ⓕ Ⓢ Ⓢ

Muscle Group Focus ____________   Weight ______   Date/Time ______

Stretch ◯   Warm-Up ____________

Strength Training

Exercise		Set 1	Set 2	Set 3	Set 4	Set 5	Set 6
	Reps						
	Weight						
	Reps						
	Weight						
	Reps						
	Weight						
	Reps						
	Weight						
	Reps						
	Weight						
	Reps						
	Weight						
	Reps						
	Weight						
	Reps						
	Weight						
	Reps						
	Weight						
	Reps						
	Weight						

Cardio

Exercise	Calories	Distance	Time

Water Intake ____________

Cooldown ____________

Feeling ☆ ☆ ☆ ☆ ☆

Notes

Today's Goal _______________ Ⓜ Ⓣ Ⓦ Ⓣ Ⓕ ⬤S ⬤S

Muscle Group Focus _______________   Weight ________   Date/Time __________

Stretch ◯   Warm-Up ____

Strength Training

Exercise		Set 1	Set 2	Set 3	Set 4	Set 5	Set 6
	Reps						
	Weight						
	Reps						
	Weight						
	Reps						
	Weight						
	Reps						
	Weight						
	Reps						
	Weight						
	Reps						
	Weight						
	Reps						
	Weight						
	Reps						
	Weight						
	Reps						
	Weight						
	Reps						
	Weight						

Cardio

Exercise	Calories	Distance	Time

Water Intake __________________

Cooldown __________________

Feeling ☆ ☆ ☆ ☆ ☆

Notes

Today's Goal   ____________________   Ⓜ Ⓣ Ⓦ Ⓣ Ⓕ ⬤ ⬤

Muscle Group Focus ________________   Weight ________   Date/Time _________

Stretch ◯   Warm-Up _____________________________________

Strength Training

Exercise		Set 1	Set 2	Set 3	Set 4	Set 5	Set 6
	Reps						
	Weight						
	Reps						
	Weight						
	Reps						
	Weight						
	Reps						
	Weight						
	Reps						
	Weight						
	Reps						
	Weight						
	Reps						
	Weight						
	Reps						
	Weight						
	Reps						
	Weight						
	Reps						
	Weight						

Cardio

Exercise	Calories	Distance	Time

Water Intake ____________________

Cooldown ____________________

Feeling ☆ ☆ ☆ ☆ ☆

Notes

Today's Goal ___________   (M) (T) (W) (T) (F) (S) (S)

Muscle Group Focus ___________   Weight _______   Date/Time _______

Stretch ◯   Warm-Up _______________________________

Strength Training

Exercise		Set 1	Set 2	Set 3	Set 4	Set 5	Set 6
	Reps						
	Weight						
	Reps						
	Weight						
	Reps						
	Weight						
	Reps						
	Weight						
	Reps						
	Weight						
	Reps						
	Weight						
	Reps						
	Weight						
	Reps						
	Weight						
	Reps						
	Weight						
	Reps						
	Weight						

Cardio

Exercise	Calories	Distance	Time

Water Intake _______________

Cooldown _______________

Feeling ☆ ☆ ☆ ☆ ☆

Notes

Today's Goal ___________ (M) (T) (W) (T) (F) (S) (S)

Muscle Group Focus ___________   Weight _______   Date/Time _______

Stretch ◯   Warm-Up ___________

Strength Training

Exercise		Set 1	Set 2	Set 3	Set 4	Set 5	Set 6
	Reps						
	Weight						
	Reps						
	Weight						
	Reps						
	Weight						
	Reps						
	Weight						
	Reps						
	Weight						
	Reps						
	Weight						
	Reps						
	Weight						
	Reps						
	Weight						
	Reps						
	Weight						
	Reps						
	Weight						

Cardio

Exercise	Calories	Distance	Time

Water Intake ___________

Cooldown ___________

Feeling ☆ ☆ ☆ ☆ ☆

Notes

Today's Goal ____________________ Ⓜ Ⓣ Ⓦ Ⓣ Ⓕ ⚫S ⚫S

Muscle Group Focus ____________ Weight ______ Date/Time __________

Stretch ◯ Warm-Up ____________________________

Strength Training

Exercise		Set 1	Set 2	Set 3	Set 4	Set 5	Set 6
	Reps						
	Weight						
	Reps						
	Weight						
	Reps						
	Weight						
	Reps						
	Weight						
	Reps						
	Weight						
	Reps						
	Weight						
	Reps						
	Weight						
	Reps						
	Weight						
	Reps						
	Weight						
	Reps						
	Weight						

Cardio

Exercise	Calories	Distance	Time

Water Intake ____________________

Cooldown ____________________

Feeling ☆ ☆ ☆ ☆ ☆

Notes

Today's Goal ____________________ (M) (T) (W) (T) (F) **(S) (S)**

Muscle Group Focus ____________________ Weight ________ Date/Time __________

Stretch ◯   Warm-Up ____

Strength Training

Exercise		Set 1	Set 2	Set 3	Set 4	Set 5	Set 6
	Reps						
	Weight						
	Reps						
	Weight						
	Reps						
	Weight						
	Reps						
	Weight						
	Reps						
	Weight						
	Reps						
	Weight						
	Reps						
	Weight						
	Reps						
	Weight						
	Reps						
	Weight						
	Reps						
	Weight						

Cardio

Exercise	Calories	Distance	Time

Water Intake ________________________

Cooldown ________________________

Feeling ☆ ☆ ☆ ☆ ☆

Notes

Today's Goal

Today's Goal ___________________ (M) (T) (W) (T) (F) (S) (S)

Muscle Group Focus ________________   Weight _________   Date/Time ___________

Stretch ◯   Warm-Up ____

Strength Training

Exercise		Set 1	Set 2	Set 3	Set 4	Set 5	Set 6
	Reps						
	Weight						
	Reps						
	Weight						
	Reps						
	Weight						
	Reps						
	Weight						
	Reps						
	Weight						
	Reps						
	Weight						
	Reps						
	Weight						
	Reps						
	Weight						
	Reps						
	Weight						

Cardio

Exercise	Calories	Distance	Time

Water Intake ___________________

Cooldown ___________________

Feeling ☆ ☆ ☆ ☆ ☆

Notes

Today's Goal

Today's Goal _______________ Ⓜ Ⓣ Ⓦ Ⓣ Ⓕ ⬤S ⬤S

Muscle Group Focus _______________ Weight _______ Date/Time _______

Stretch ◯   Warm-Up _______________

Strength Training

Exercise		Set 1	Set 2	Set 3	Set 4	Set 5	Set 6
	Reps						
	Weight						
	Reps						
	Weight						
	Reps						
	Weight						
	Reps						
	Weight						
	Reps						
	Weight						
	Reps						
	Weight						
	Reps						
	Weight						
	Reps						
	Weight						
	Reps						
	Weight						
	Reps						
	Weight						

Cardio

Exercise	Calories	Distance	Time

Water Intake _______________

Cooldown _______________

Feeling ☆ ☆ ☆ ☆ ☆

Notes

Today's Goal _______________ (M) (T) (W) (T) (F) (S) (S)

Muscle Group Focus _______________   Weight _______   Date/Time _______________

Stretch ◯   Warm-Up ____

Strength Training

Exercise		Set 1	Set 2	Set 3	Set 4	Set 5	Set 6
	Reps						
	Weight						
	Reps						
	Weight						
	Reps						
	Weight						
	Reps						
	Weight						
	Reps						
	Weight						
	Reps						
	Weight						
	Reps						
	Weight						
	Reps						
	Weight						
	Reps						
	Weight						

Cardio

Exercise	Calories	Distance	Time

Water Intake _______________

Cooldown _______________

Feeling ☆ ☆ ☆ ☆ ☆

Notes

Today's Goal _______________ (M)(T)(W)(T)(F)(S)(S)

Muscle Group Focus _______________ Weight ________ Date/Time _________

Stretch ○ Warm-Up _______________________________________

Strength Training

Exercise		Set 1	Set 2	Set 3	Set 4	Set 5	Set 6
	Reps						
	Weight						
	Reps						
	Weight						
	Reps						
	Weight						
	Reps						
	Weight						
	Reps						
	Weight						
	Reps						
	Weight						
	Reps						
	Weight						
	Reps						
	Weight						
	Reps						
	Weight						

Cardio

Exercise	Calories	Distance	Time

Water Intake _______________

Cooldown _______________

Feeling ☆ ☆ ☆ ☆ ☆

Notes

Today's Goal ______________ Ⓜ Ⓣ Ⓦ Ⓣ Ⓕ ⬤S ⬤S

Muscle Group Focus ______________   Weight ________   Date/Time __________

Stretch ◯   Warm-Up ________________________________

Strength Training

Exercise		Set 1	Set 2	Set 3	Set 4	Set 5	Set 6
	Reps						
	Weight						
	Reps						
	Weight						
	Reps						
	Weight						
	Reps						
	Weight						
	Reps						
	Weight						
	Reps						
	Weight						
	Reps						
	Weight						
	Reps						
	Weight						
	Reps						
	Weight						
	Reps						
	Weight						

Cardio

Exercise	Calories	Distance	Time

Water Intake ________________

Cooldown ________________

Feeling ☆ ☆ ☆ ☆ ☆

Notes

Today's Goal ___________________ Ⓜ Ⓣ Ⓦ Ⓣ Ⓕ ⚫S ⚫S

Muscle Group Focus _______________ Weight _______ Date/Time _________

Stretch ◯   Warm-Up _________________________________

Strength Training

Exercise		Set 1	Set 2	Set 3	Set 4	Set 5	Set 6
	Reps						
	Weight						
	Reps						
	Weight						
	Reps						
	Weight						
	Reps						
	Weight						
	Reps						
	Weight						
	Reps						
	Weight						
	Reps						
	Weight						
	Reps						
	Weight						
	Reps						
	Weight						
	Reps						
	Weight						

Cardio

Exercise	Calories	Distance	Time

Water Intake _________________

Cooldown _________________

Feeling ☆ ☆ ☆ ☆ ☆

Notes

Today's Goal ______________________ Ⓜ Ⓣ Ⓦ Ⓣ Ⓕ ⬤S ⬤S

Muscle Group Focus ______________ Weight ________ Date/Time __________

Stretch ◯   Warm-Up ____

Strength Training

Exercise		Set 1	Set 2	Set 3	Set 4	Set 5	Set 6
	Reps						
	Weight						
	Reps						
	Weight						
	Reps						
	Weight						
	Reps						
	Weight						
	Reps						
	Weight						
	Reps						
	Weight						
	Reps						
	Weight						
	Reps						
	Weight						

Cardio

Exercise	Calories	Distance	Time

Water Intake ___________________

Cooldown ___________________

Feeling ☆ ☆ ☆ ☆ ☆

Notes

Today's Goal _______________ Ⓜ Ⓣ Ⓦ Ⓣ Ⓕ ⬤S ⬤S

Muscle Group Focus _______________   Weight _______   Date/Time _______

Stretch ◯   Warm-Up _________________________________

Strength Training

Exercise		Set 1	Set 2	Set 3	Set 4	Set 5	Set 6
	Reps						
	Weight						
	Reps						
	Weight						
	Reps						
	Weight						
	Reps						
	Weight						
	Reps						
	Weight						
	Reps						
	Weight						
	Reps						
	Weight						
	Reps						
	Weight						
	Reps						
	Weight						

Cardio

Exercise	Calories	Distance	Time

Water Intake _________________

Cooldown _________________

Feeling ☆ ☆ ☆ ☆ ☆

Notes

Today's Goal ___________   Ⓜ Ⓣ Ⓦ Ⓣ Ⓕ ⚫S ⚫S

Muscle Group Focus ___________   Weight _______   Date/Time ___________

Stretch ◯   Warm-Up ___________________________________

Strength Training

Exercise		Set 1	Set 2	Set 3	Set 4	Set 5	Set 6
	Reps						
	Weight						
	Reps						
	Weight						
	Reps						
	Weight						
	Reps						
	Weight						
	Reps						
	Weight						
	Reps						
	Weight						
	Reps						
	Weight						
	Reps						
	Weight						
	Reps						
	Weight						
	Reps						
	Weight						

Cardio

Exercise	Calories	Distance	Time

Water Intake ___________

Cooldown ___________

Feeling ☆ ☆ ☆ ☆ ☆

Notes

Today's Goal ______________________   (M) (T) (W) (T) (F) **(S) (S)**

Muscle Group Focus ______________   Weight ________   Date/Time __________

Stretch ◯   Warm-Up ____

Strength Training

Exercise		Set 1	Set 2	Set 3	Set 4	Set 5	Set 6
	Reps						
	Weight						
	Reps						
	Weight						
	Reps						
	Weight						
	Reps						
	Weight						
	Reps						
	Weight						
	Reps						
	Weight						
	Reps						
	Weight						
	Reps						
	Weight						
	Reps						
	Weight						
	Reps						
	Weight						

Cardio

Exercise	Calories	Distance	Time

Water Intake ________________________

Cooldown ________________________

Feeling ☆ ☆ ☆ ☆ ☆

Notes

Today's Goal

Today's Goal _________________ (M) (T) (W) (T) (F) (S) (S)

Muscle Group Focus _______________ Weight ________ Date/Time __________

Stretch ◯ Warm-Up _____________________________________

Strength Training

Exercise		Set 1	Set 2	Set 3	Set 4	Set 5	Set 6
	Reps						
	Weight						
	Reps						
	Weight						
	Reps						
	Weight						
	Reps						
	Weight						
	Reps						
	Weight						
	Reps						
	Weight						
	Reps						
	Weight						
	Reps						
	Weight						
	Reps						
	Weight						

Cardio

Exercise	Calories	Distance	Time

Water Intake ____________________

Cooldown __________________

Feeling ☆ ☆ ☆ ☆ ☆

Notes

Today's Goal _______________   (M) (T) (W) (T) (F) (S) (S)

Muscle Group Focus _______________   Weight ________   Date/Time __________

Stretch ◯   Warm-Up ____

Strength Training

Exercise		Set 1	Set 2	Set 3	Set 4	Set 5	Set 6
	Reps						
	Weight						
	Reps						
	Weight						
	Reps						
	Weight						
	Reps						
	Weight						
	Reps						
	Weight						
	Reps						
	Weight						
	Reps						
	Weight						
	Reps						
	Weight						

Cardio

Exercise	Calories	Distance	Time

Water Intake _______________________

Cooldown _______________________

Feeling ☆ ☆ ☆ ☆ ☆

Notes

Today's Goal ________________   Ⓜ Ⓣ Ⓦ Ⓣ Ⓕ ⬤S ⬤S

Muscle Group Focus ____________   Weight ________   Date/Time __________

Stretch ◯   Warm-Up ________________________________

Strength Training

Exercise		Set 1	Set 2	Set 3	Set 4	Set 5	Set 6
	Reps						
	Weight						
	Reps						
	Weight						
	Reps						
	Weight						
	Reps						
	Weight						
	Reps						
	Weight						
	Reps						
	Weight						
	Reps						
	Weight						
	Reps						
	Weight						
	Reps						
	Weight						
	Reps						
	Weight						

Cardio

Exercise	Calories	Distance	Time

Water Intake __________________

Cooldown __________________

Feeling ☆ ☆ ☆ ☆ ☆

Notes

Today's Goal ___________________ (M) (T) (W) (T) (F) (S) (S)

Muscle Group Focus _______________   Weight _______   Date/Time _______

Stretch ◯   Warm-Up ___________________________________

Strength Training

Exercise		Set 1	Set 2	Set 3	Set 4	Set 5	Set 6
	Reps						
	Weight						
	Reps						
	Weight						
	Reps						
	Weight						
	Reps						
	Weight						
	Reps						
	Weight						
	Reps						
	Weight						
	Reps						
	Weight						
	Reps						
	Weight						
	Reps						
	Weight						
	Reps						
	Weight						

Cardio

Exercise	Calories	Distance	Time

Water Intake _______________

Cooldown _______________

Feeling ☆ ☆ ☆ ☆ ☆

Notes

Today's Goal ___________ Ⓜ Ⓣ Ⓦ Ⓣ Ⓕ ⬤S ⬤S

Muscle Group Focus ___________   Weight _______   Date/Time __________

Stretch ◯   Warm-Up _________________________________

Strength Training

Exercise		Set 1	Set 2	Set 3	Set 4	Set 5	Set 6
	Reps						
	Weight						
	Reps						
	Weight						
	Reps						
	Weight						
	Reps						
	Weight						
	Reps						
	Weight						
	Reps						
	Weight						
	Reps						
	Weight						
	Reps						
	Weight						
	Reps						
	Weight						
	Reps						
	Weight						

Cardio

Exercise	Calories	Distance	Time

Water Intake ___________

Cooldown ___________

Feeling ☆ ☆ ☆ ☆ ☆

Notes

Today's Goal _______________   (M) (T) (W) (T) (F) (S) (S)

Muscle Group Focus _______________   Weight _______   Date/Time _______

Stretch ◯   Warm-Up _________________________

Strength Training

Exercise		Set 1	Set 2	Set 3	Set 4	Set 5	Set 6
	Reps						
	Weight						
	Reps						
	Weight						
	Reps						
	Weight						
	Reps						
	Weight						
	Reps						
	Weight						
	Reps						
	Weight						
	Reps						
	Weight						
	Reps						
	Weight						
	Reps						
	Weight						
	Reps						
	Weight						

Cardio

Exercise	Calories	Distance	Time

Water Intake _________________

Cooldown _________________

Feeling ☆ ☆ ☆ ☆ ☆

Notes

Today's Goal ___________________ (M) (T) (W) (T) (F) (S) (S)

Muscle Group Focus ________________ Weight ________ Date/Time __________

Stretch ◯   Warm-Up ________________________________

Strength Training

Exercise		Set 1	Set 2	Set 3	Set 4	Set 5	Set 6
	Reps						
	Weight						
	Reps						
	Weight						
	Reps						
	Weight						
	Reps						
	Weight						
	Reps						
	Weight						
	Reps						
	Weight						
	Reps						
	Weight						
	Reps						
	Weight						
	Reps						
	Weight						

Cardio

Exercise	Calories	Distance	Time

Water Intake ________________

Cooldown ________________

Feeling ☆ ☆ ☆ ☆ ☆

Notes

Today's Goal ______________ Ⓜ Ⓣ Ⓦ Ⓣ Ⓕ Ⓢ Ⓢ

Muscle Group Focus ______________ Weight ______ Date/Time ______

Stretch ◯   Warm-Up ______________________________

Strength Training

Exercise		Set 1	Set 2	Set 3	Set 4	Set 5	Set 6
	Reps						
	Weight						
	Reps						
	Weight						
	Reps						
	Weight						
	Reps						
	Weight						
	Reps						
	Weight						
	Reps						
	Weight						
	Reps						
	Weight						
	Reps						
	Weight						
	Reps						
	Weight						

Cardio

Exercise	Calories	Distance	Time

Water Intake ______________

Cooldown ______________

Feeling ☆ ☆ ☆ ☆ ☆

Notes

Today's Goal _______________   Ⓜ Ⓣ Ⓦ Ⓣ Ⓕ Ⓢ Ⓢ

Muscle Group Focus _____________   Weight _______   Date/Time _________

Stretch ◯   Warm-Up ____

Strength Training

Exercise		Set 1	Set 2	Set 3	Set 4	Set 5	Set 6
	Reps						
	Weight						
	Reps						
	Weight						
	Reps						
	Weight						
	Reps						
	Weight						
	Reps						
	Weight						
	Reps						
	Weight						
	Reps						
	Weight						
	Reps						
	Weight						
	Reps						
	Weight						

Cardio

Exercise	Calories	Distance	Time

Water Intake _________________

Cooldown _________________

Feeling ☆ ☆ ☆ ☆ ☆

Notes

Today's Goal _____________ Ⓜ Ⓣ Ⓦ Ⓣ Ⓕ ⬤S ⬤S

Muscle Group Focus _____________   Weight _______   Date/Time _________

Stretch ◯   Warm-Up _______________________________

Strength Training

Exercise		Set 1	Set 2	Set 3	Set 4	Set 5	Set 6
	Reps						
	Weight						
	Reps						
	Weight						
	Reps						
	Weight						
	Reps						
	Weight						
	Reps						
	Weight						
	Reps						
	Weight						
	Reps						
	Weight						
	Reps						
	Weight						
	Reps						
	Weight						
	Reps						
	Weight						

Cardio

Exercise	Calories	Distance	Time

Water Intake _______________

Cooldown _______________

Feeling ☆ ☆ ☆ ☆ ☆

Notes

Today's Goal ______________ (M) (T) (W) (T) (F) (S) (S)

Muscle Group Focus ______________   Weight ________   Date/Time ____________

Stretch ◯   Warm-Up ____

Strength Training

Exercise		Set 1	Set 2	Set 3	Set 4	Set 5	Set 6
	Reps						
	Weight						
	Reps						
	Weight						
	Reps						
	Weight						
	Reps						
	Weight						
	Reps						
	Weight						
	Reps						
	Weight						
	Reps						
	Weight						
	Reps						
	Weight						
	Reps						
	Weight						
	Reps						
	Weight						

Cardio

Exercise	Calories	Distance	Time

Water Intake ________________

Cooldown ________________

Feeling ☆ ☆ ☆ ☆ ☆

Notes

Today's Goal ______________   Ⓜ Ⓣ Ⓦ Ⓣ Ⓕ Ⓢ Ⓢ

Muscle Group Focus ______________   Weight ________   Date/Time ________

Stretch ◯   Warm-Up ________________________

Strength Training

Exercise		Set 1	Set 2	Set 3	Set 4	Set 5	Set 6
	Reps						
	Weight						
	Reps						
	Weight						
	Reps						
	Weight						
	Reps						
	Weight						
	Reps						
	Weight						
	Reps						
	Weight						
	Reps						
	Weight						
	Reps						
	Weight						
	Reps						
	Weight						
	Reps						
	Weight						

Cardio

Exercise	Calories	Distance	Time

Water Intake ________________

Cooldown ________________

Feeling ☆ ☆ ☆ ☆ ☆

Notes

Today's Goal

Today's Goal __________________ (M) (T) (W) (T) (F) (S) (S)

Muscle Group Focus ______________ Weight _______ Date/Time __________

Stretch ◯   Warm-Up ____

Strength Training

Exercise		Set 1	Set 2	Set 3	Set 4	Set 5	Set 6
	Reps						
	Weight						
	Reps						
	Weight						
	Reps						
	Weight						
	Reps						
	Weight						
	Reps						
	Weight						
	Reps						
	Weight						
	Reps						
	Weight						
	Reps						
	Weight						
	Reps						
	Weight						

Cardio

Exercise	Calories	Distance	Time

Water Intake ________________________

Cooldown ______________________

Feeling ☆ ☆ ☆ ☆ ☆

Notes

Today's Goal ______________   (M) (T) (W) (T) (F) (S) (S)

Muscle Group Focus ______________   Weight ________   Date/Time __________

Stretch ◯   Warm-Up ___________________________

Strength Training

Exercise		Set 1	Set 2	Set 3	Set 4	Set 5	Set 6
	Reps						
	Weight						
	Reps						
	Weight						
	Reps						
	Weight						
	Reps						
	Weight						
	Reps						
	Weight						
	Reps						
	Weight						
	Reps						
	Weight						
	Reps						
	Weight						
	Reps						
	Weight						
	Reps						
	Weight						

Cardio

Exercise	Calories	Distance	Time

Water Intake ___________________

Cooldown ___________________

Feeling ☆ ☆ ☆ ☆ ☆

Notes

Today's Goal _______________   Ⓜ Ⓣ Ⓦ Ⓣ Ⓕ ⬤S ⬤S

Muscle Group Focus _______________   Weight _______   Date/Time _______

Stretch ◯   Warm-Up _______________________________

Strength Training

Exercise		Set 1	Set 2	Set 3	Set 4	Set 5	Set 6
	Reps						
	Weight						
	Reps						
	Weight						
	Reps						
	Weight						
	Reps						
	Weight						
	Reps						
	Weight						
	Reps						
	Weight						
	Reps						
	Weight						
	Reps						
	Weight						
	Reps						
	Weight						
	Reps						
	Weight						

Cardio

Exercise	Calories	Distance	Time

Water Intake _______________

Cooldown _______________

Feeling ☆ ☆ ☆ ☆ ☆

Notes

Today's Goal ______________ (M) (T) (W) (T) (F) (S) (S)

Muscle Group Focus ______________   Weight _______   Date/Time _______

Stretch ◯   Warm-Up _______________________________

Strength Training

Exercise		Set 1	Set 2	Set 3	Set 4	Set 5	Set 6
	Reps						
	Weight						
	Reps						
	Weight						
	Reps						
	Weight						
	Reps						
	Weight						
	Reps						
	Weight						
	Reps						
	Weight						
	Reps						
	Weight						
	Reps						
	Weight						
	Reps						
	Weight						
	Reps						
	Weight						

Cardio

Exercise	Calories	Distance	Time

Water Intake _______________

Cooldown _______________

Feeling ☆ ☆ ☆ ☆ ☆

Notes

Today's Goal ______________   M T W T F **S** **S**

Muscle Group Focus ______________   Weight ________   Date/Time ____________

Stretch ◯   Warm-Up ____

Strength Training

Exercise		Set 1	Set 2	Set 3	Set 4	Set 5	Set 6
	Reps						
	Weight						
	Reps						
	Weight						
	Reps						
	Weight						
	Reps						
	Weight						
	Reps						
	Weight						
	Reps						
	Weight						
	Reps						
	Weight						
	Reps						
	Weight						
	Reps						
	Weight						
	Reps						
	Weight						

Cardio

Exercise	Calories	Distance	Time

Water Intake ________________

Cooldown ________________

Feeling ☆ ☆ ☆ ☆ ☆

Notes

Today's Goal ___________ Ⓜ Ⓣ Ⓦ Ⓣ Ⓕ Ⓢ Ⓢ

Muscle Group Focus ___________ Weight ______ Date/Time ______

Stretch ◯   Warm-Up ___________

Strength Training

Exercise		Set 1	Set 2	Set 3	Set 4	Set 5	Set 6
	Reps						
	Weight						
	Reps						
	Weight						
	Reps						
	Weight						
	Reps						
	Weight						
	Reps						
	Weight						
	Reps						
	Weight						
	Reps						
	Weight						
	Reps						
	Weight						
	Reps						
	Weight						
	Reps						
	Weight						

Cardio

Exercise	Calories	Distance	Time

Water Intake ___________

Cooldown ___________

Feeling ☆ ☆ ☆ ☆ ☆

Notes

Today's Goal __________   Ⓜ Ⓣ Ⓦ Ⓣ Ⓕ Ⓢ Ⓢ

Muscle Group Focus __________   Weight __________   Date/Time __________

Stretch ◯   Warm-Up __________

Strength Training

Exercise		Set 1	Set 2	Set 3	Set 4	Set 5	Set 6
	Reps						
	Weight						
	Reps						
	Weight						
	Reps						
	Weight						
	Reps						
	Weight						
	Reps						
	Weight						
	Reps						
	Weight						
	Reps						
	Weight						
	Reps						
	Weight						
	Reps						
	Weight						
	Reps						
	Weight						

Cardio

Exercise	Calories	Distance	Time

Water Intake __________

Cooldown __________

Feeling ☆ ☆ ☆ ☆ ☆

Notes

Today's Goal ____________________   (M) (T) (W) (T) (F) (S) (S)

Muscle Group Focus ____________   Weight ________   Date/Time __________

Stretch ◯   Warm-Up ____________________________________

Strength Training

Exercise		Set 1	Set 2	Set 3	Set 4	Set 5	Set 6
	Reps						
	Weight						
	Reps						
	Weight						
	Reps						
	Weight						
	Reps						
	Weight						
	Reps						
	Weight						
	Reps						
	Weight						
	Reps						
	Weight						
	Reps						
	Weight						
	Reps						
	Weight						
	Reps						
	Weight						

Cardio

Exercise	Calories	Distance	Time

Water Intake ____________________

Cooldown ____________________

Feeling ☆ ☆ ☆ ☆ ☆

Notes

Today's Goal ___________ Ⓜ Ⓣ Ⓦ Ⓣ Ⓕ **Ⓢ Ⓢ**

Muscle Group Focus ___________   Weight _______   Date/Time _________

Stretch ◯   Warm-Up ___________________________

Strength Training

Exercise		Set 1	Set 2	Set 3	Set 4	Set 5	Set 6
	Reps						
	Weight						
	Reps						
	Weight						
	Reps						
	Weight						
	Reps						
	Weight						
	Reps						
	Weight						
	Reps						
	Weight						
	Reps						
	Weight						
	Reps						
	Weight						
	Reps						
	Weight						
	Reps						
	Weight						

Cardio

Exercise	Calories	Distance	Time

Water Intake ___________

Cooldown ___________

Feeling ☆ ☆ ☆ ☆ ☆

Notes

Today's Goal   _________________   (M) (T) (W) (T) (F) **(S)** **(S)**

Muscle Group Focus   _________________   Weight _________   Date/Time _________

Stretch ◯   Warm-Up   ____

Strength Training

Exercise		Set 1	Set 2	Set 3	Set 4	Set 5	Set 6
	Reps						
	Weight						
	Reps						
	Weight						
	Reps						
	Weight						
	Reps						
	Weight						
	Reps						
	Weight						
	Reps						
	Weight						
	Reps						
	Weight						
	Reps						
	Weight						
	Reps						
	Weight						
	Reps						
	Weight						

Cardio

Exercise	Calories	Distance	Time

Water Intake   _________________

Cooldown   _________________

Feeling ☆ ☆ ☆ ☆ ☆

Notes

Today's Goal ___________ (M) (T) (W) (T) (F) (S) (S)

Muscle Group Focus ___________   Weight _______   Date/Time ___________

Stretch ◯   Warm-Up ___________________________________

Strength Training

Exercise		Set 1	Set 2	Set 3	Set 4	Set 5	Set 6
	Reps						
	Weight						
	Reps						
	Weight						
	Reps						
	Weight						
	Reps						
	Weight						
	Reps						
	Weight						
	Reps						
	Weight						
	Reps						
	Weight						
	Reps						
	Weight						
	Reps						
	Weight						
	Reps						
	Weight						

Cardio

Exercise	Calories	Distance	Time

Water Intake ___________

Cooldown ___________

Feeling ☆ ☆ ☆ ☆ ☆

Notes

Today's Goal ___________________ Ⓜ Ⓣ Ⓦ Ⓣ Ⓕ ● ●

Muscle Group Focus ________________ Weight ________ Date/Time __________

Stretch ◯   Warm-Up ____

Strength Training

Exercise		Set 1	Set 2	Set 3	Set 4	Set 5	Set 6
_______	Reps						
	Weight						
_______	Reps						
	Weight						
_______	Reps						
	Weight						
_______	Reps						
	Weight						
_______	Reps						
	Weight						
_______	Reps						
	Weight						
_______	Reps						
	Weight						
_______	Reps						
	Weight						
_______	Reps						
	Weight						

Cardio

Exercise	Calories	Distance	Time
_______			
_______			
_______			

Water Intake ________________

Cooldown ________________

Feeling ☆ ☆ ☆ ☆ ☆

Notes

Today's Goal ________________ Ⓜ Ⓣ Ⓦ Ⓣ Ⓕ ⬤ ⬤

Muscle Group Focus ________________   Weight ________   Date/Time ____________

Stretch ◯   Warm-Up ____

Strength Training

Exercise		Set 1	Set 2	Set 3	Set 4	Set 5	Set 6
	Reps						
	Weight						
	Reps						
	Weight						
	Reps						
	Weight						
	Reps						
	Weight						
	Reps						
	Weight						
	Reps						
	Weight						
	Reps						
	Weight						
	Reps						
	Weight						
	Reps						
	Weight						

Cardio

Exercise	Calories	Distance	Time

Water Intake ________________

Cooldown ________________

Feeling ☆ ☆ ☆ ☆ ☆

Notes

Today's Goal ________________   Ⓜ Ⓣ Ⓦ Ⓣ Ⓕ ⚫ ⚫

Muscle Group Focus ________________   Weight ________   Date/Time ________

Stretch ◯   Warm-Up ________________________________

Strength Training

Exercise		Set 1	Set 2	Set 3	Set 4	Set 5	Set 6
	Reps						
	Weight						
	Reps						
	Weight						
	Reps						
	Weight						
	Reps						
	Weight						
	Reps						
	Weight						
	Reps						
	Weight						
	Reps						
	Weight						
	Reps						
	Weight						
	Reps						
	Weight						
	Reps						
	Weight						

Cardio

Exercise	Calories	Distance	Time

Water Intake ________________

Cooldown ________________

Feeling ☆ ☆ ☆ ☆ ☆

Notes

Today's Goal ___________   Ⓜ Ⓣ Ⓦ Ⓣ Ⓕ ⬤S ⬤S

Muscle Group Focus ___________   Weight _______   Date/Time _______

Stretch ◯   Warm-Up ___________________________

Strength Training

Exercise		Set 1	Set 2	Set 3	Set 4	Set 5	Set 6
	Reps						
	Weight						
	Reps						
	Weight						
	Reps						
	Weight						
	Reps						
	Weight						
	Reps						
	Weight						
	Reps						
	Weight						
	Reps						
	Weight						
	Reps						
	Weight						
	Reps						
	Weight						

Cardio

Exercise	Calories	Distance	Time

Water Intake ___________________

Cooldown ___________________

Feeling ☆ ☆ ☆ ☆ ☆

Notes

Today's Goal ________________ (M) (T) (W) (T) (F) (S) (S)

Muscle Group Focus ______________   Weight ________   Date/Time __________

Stretch ◯   Warm-Up ____

Strength Training

Exercise		Set 1	Set 2	Set 3	Set 4	Set 5	Set 6
	Reps						
	Weight						
	Reps						
	Weight						
	Reps						
	Weight						
	Reps						
	Weight						
	Reps						
	Weight						
	Reps						
	Weight						
	Reps						
	Weight						
	Reps						
	Weight						
	Reps						
	Weight						
	Reps						
	Weight						

Cardio

Exercise	Calories	Distance	Time

Water Intake ____________________

Cooldown ____________________

Feeling ☆ ☆ ☆ ☆ ☆

Notes

____

Today's Goal ____________ Ⓜ Ⓣ Ⓦ Ⓣ Ⓕ Ⓢ Ⓢ

Muscle Group Focus ____________   Weight ________   Date/Time ________

Stretch ◯   Warm-Up ________________________________

Strength Training

Exercise		Set 1	Set 2	Set 3	Set 4	Set 5	Set 6
	Reps						
	Weight						
	Reps						
	Weight						
	Reps						
	Weight						
	Reps						
	Weight						
	Reps						
	Weight						
	Reps						
	Weight						
	Reps						
	Weight						
	Reps						
	Weight						
	Reps						
	Weight						
	Reps						
	Weight						

Cardio

Exercise	Calories	Distance	Time

Water Intake ________________

Cooldown ________________

Feeling ☆ ☆ ☆ ☆ ☆

Notes

Today's Goal _______________   (M) (T) (W) (T) (F) (S) (S)

Muscle Group Focus _______________   Weight _______   Date/Time _______

Stretch ◯   Warm-Up _______________________________

Strength Training

Exercise		Set 1	Set 2	Set 3	Set 4	Set 5	Set 6
	Reps						
	Weight						
	Reps						
	Weight						
	Reps						
	Weight						
	Reps						
	Weight						
	Reps						
	Weight						
	Reps						
	Weight						
	Reps						
	Weight						
	Reps						
	Weight						
	Reps						
	Weight						
	Reps						
	Weight						

Cardio

Exercise	Calories	Distance	Time

Water Intake _______________

Cooldown _______________

Feeling ☆ ☆ ☆ ☆ ☆

Notes

Today's Goal ______________ Ⓜ Ⓣ Ⓦ Ⓣ Ⓕ ● ●

Muscle Group Focus ______________ Weight ________ Date/Time __________

Stretch ◯ Warm-Up ________________________________

Strength Training

Exercise		Set 1	Set 2	Set 3	Set 4	Set 5	Set 6
	Reps						
	Weight						
	Reps						
	Weight						
	Reps						
	Weight						
	Reps						
	Weight						
	Reps						
	Weight						
	Reps						
	Weight						
	Reps						
	Weight						
	Reps						
	Weight						
	Reps						
	Weight						
	Reps						
	Weight						

Cardio

Exercise	Calories	Distance	Time

Water Intake ________________

Cooldown ________________

Feeling ☆ ☆ ☆ ☆ ☆

Notes

Today's Goal ____________________   (M) (T) (W) (T) (F) (S) (S)

Muscle Group Focus ____________ Weight ______ Date/Time __________

Stretch ◯   Warm-Up ________________________________

Strength Training

Exercise		Set 1	Set 2	Set 3	Set 4	Set 5	Set 6
	Reps						
	Weight						
	Reps						
	Weight						
	Reps						
	Weight						
	Reps						
	Weight						
	Reps						
	Weight						
	Reps						
	Weight						
	Reps						
	Weight						
	Reps						
	Weight						
	Reps						
	Weight						
	Reps						
	Weight						

Cardio

Exercise	Calories	Distance	Time

Water Intake ________________

Cooldown ________________

Feeling ☆ ☆ ☆ ☆ ☆

Notes

Today's Goal ________________ Ⓜ Ⓣ Ⓦ Ⓣ Ⓕ **S** **S**

Muscle Group Focus ________________   Weight ________   Date/Time ________

Stretch ◯   Warm-Up ________________________________

Strength Training

Exercise		Set 1	Set 2	Set 3	Set 4	Set 5	Set 6
	Reps						
	Weight						
	Reps						
	Weight						
	Reps						
	Weight						
	Reps						
	Weight						
	Reps						
	Weight						
	Reps						
	Weight						
	Reps						
	Weight						
	Reps						
	Weight						
	Reps						
	Weight						

Cardio

Exercise	Calories	Distance	Time

Water Intake ________________

Cooldown ________________

Feeling ☆ ☆ ☆ ☆ ☆

Notes

Today's Goal _______________   (M) (T) (W) (T) (F) (S) (S)

Muscle Group Focus _______________   Weight _______   Date/Time _______

Stretch ◯   Warm-Up _______________________________

Strength Training

Exercise		Set 1	Set 2	Set 3	Set 4	Set 5	Set 6
	Reps						
	Weight						
	Reps						
	Weight						
	Reps						
	Weight						
	Reps						
	Weight						
	Reps						
	Weight						
	Reps						
	Weight						
	Reps						
	Weight						
	Reps						
	Weight						
	Reps						
	Weight						

Cardio

Exercise	Calories	Distance	Time

Water Intake _______________

Cooldown _______________

Feeling ☆ ☆ ☆ ☆ ☆

Notes

Today's Goal ________________   (M) (T) (W) (T) (F) (S) (S)

Muscle Group Focus ________________   Weight ________   Date/Time ____________

Stretch ◯   Warm-Up ____

Strength Training

Exercise		Set 1	Set 2	Set 3	Set 4	Set 5	Set 6
	Reps						
	Weight						
	Reps						
	Weight						
	Reps						
	Weight						
	Reps						
	Weight						
	Reps						
	Weight						
	Reps						
	Weight						
	Reps						
	Weight						
	Reps						
	Weight						
	Reps						
	Weight						
	Reps						
	Weight						

Cardio

Exercise	Calories	Distance	Time

Water Intake ________________________

Cooldown ________________________

Feeling ☆ ☆ ☆ ☆ ☆

Notes

Today's Goal ______________ Ⓜ Ⓣ Ⓦ Ⓣ Ⓕ ⚫ⓈⓈ

Muscle Group Focus ______________   Weight ________   Date/Time __________

Stretch ◯   Warm-Up ______________________________

Strength Training

Exercise		Set 1	Set 2	Set 3	Set 4	Set 5	Set 6
	Reps						
	Weight						
	Reps						
	Weight						
	Reps						
	Weight						
	Reps						
	Weight						
	Reps						
	Weight						
	Reps						
	Weight						
	Reps						
	Weight						
	Reps						
	Weight						
	Reps						
	Weight						

Cardio

Exercise	Calories	Distance	Time

Water Intake ______________

Cooldown ______________

Feeling ☆ ☆ ☆ ☆ ☆

Notes

Today's Goal _____________   Ⓜ Ⓣ Ⓦ Ⓣ Ⓕ ⬤S ⬤S

Muscle Group Focus _____________   Weight _______   Date/Time _________

Stretch ◯   Warm-Up _______________________________

Strength Training

Exercise		Set 1	Set 2	Set 3	Set 4	Set 5	Set 6
	Reps						
	Weight						
	Reps						
	Weight						
	Reps						
	Weight						
	Reps						
	Weight						
	Reps						
	Weight						
	Reps						
	Weight						
	Reps						
	Weight						
	Reps						
	Weight						
	Reps						
	Weight						

Cardio

Exercise	Calories	Distance	Time

Water Intake _______________

Cooldown _______________

Feeling ☆ ☆ ☆ ☆ ☆

Notes

Today's Goal ______________ Ⓜ Ⓣ Ⓦ Ⓣ Ⓕ ⬤ ⬤

Muscle Group Focus ______________   Weight ________   Date/Time __________

Stretch ◯   Warm-Up ___________________________________

Strength Training

Exercise		Set 1	Set 2	Set 3	Set 4	Set 5	Set 6
	Reps						
	Weight						
	Reps						
	Weight						
	Reps						
	Weight						
	Reps						
	Weight						
	Reps						
	Weight						
	Reps						
	Weight						
	Reps						
	Weight						
	Reps						
	Weight						
	Reps						
	Weight						

Cardio

Exercise	Calories	Distance	Time

Water Intake __________________

Cooldown __________________

Feeling ☆ ☆ ☆ ☆ ☆

Notes

Today's Goal ____________ Ⓜ Ⓣ Ⓦ Ⓣ Ⓕ ⬤S ⬤S

Muscle Group Focus ____________   Weight ________   Date/Time __________

Stretch ◯   Warm-Up ________________________________

Strength Training

Exercise		Set 1	Set 2	Set 3	Set 4	Set 5	Set 6
	Reps						
	Weight						
	Reps						
	Weight						
	Reps						
	Weight						
	Reps						
	Weight						
	Reps						
	Weight						
	Reps						
	Weight						
	Reps						
	Weight						
	Reps						
	Weight						
	Reps						
	Weight						

Cardio

Exercise	Calories	Distance	Time

Water Intake ________________

Cooldown ________________

Feeling ☆ ☆ ☆ ☆ ☆

Notes

Today's Goal ________________ （M）（T）（W）（T）（F）（S）（S）

Muscle Group Focus ________________   Weight ________   Date/Time ________

Stretch ◯   Warm-Up ________________________________

Strength Training

Exercise		Set 1	Set 2	Set 3	Set 4	Set 5	Set 6
	Reps						
	Weight						
	Reps						
	Weight						
	Reps						
	Weight						
	Reps						
	Weight						
	Reps						
	Weight						
	Reps						
	Weight						
	Reps						
	Weight						
	Reps						
	Weight						
	Reps						
	Weight						
	Reps						
	Weight						

Cardio

Exercise	Calories	Distance	Time

Water Intake ________________

Cooldown ________________

Feeling ☆ ☆ ☆ ☆ ☆

Notes

Today's Goal _______________ Ⓜ Ⓣ Ⓦ Ⓣ Ⓕ ⬤S ⬤S

Muscle Group Focus _____________   Weight _______   Date/Time __________

Stretch ◯   Warm-Up _______________________________________

Strength Training

Exercise		Set 1	Set 2	Set 3	Set 4	Set 5	Set 6
	Reps						
	Weight						
	Reps						
	Weight						
	Reps						
	Weight						
	Reps						
	Weight						
	Reps						
	Weight						
	Reps						
	Weight						
	Reps						
	Weight						
	Reps						
	Weight						
	Reps						
	Weight						
	Reps						
	Weight						

Cardio

Exercise	Calories	Distance	Time

Water Intake _______________

Cooldown _______________

Feeling ☆ ☆ ☆ ☆ ☆

Notes

Today's Goal _______________ Ⓜ Ⓣ Ⓦ Ⓣ Ⓕ ⬤S ⬤S

Muscle Group Focus _______________   Weight _______   Date/Time _______

Stretch ◯   Warm-Up _______________________________

Strength Training

Exercise		Set 1	Set 2	Set 3	Set 4	Set 5	Set 6
	Reps						
	Weight						
	Reps						
	Weight						
	Reps						
	Weight						
	Reps						
	Weight						
	Reps						
	Weight						
	Reps						
	Weight						
	Reps						
	Weight						
	Reps						
	Weight						
	Reps						
	Weight						

Cardio

Exercise	Calories	Distance	Time

Water Intake _______________________

Cooldown _______________________

Feeling ☆ ☆ ☆ ☆ ☆

Notes

Today's Goal ___________ (M) (T) (W) (T) (F) (S) (S)

Muscle Group Focus ___________   Weight ________   Date/Time ___________

Stretch ◯   Warm-Up ___________

Strength Training

Exercise		Set 1	Set 2	Set 3	Set 4	Set 5	Set 6
	Reps						
	Weight						
	Reps						
	Weight						
	Reps						
	Weight						
	Reps						
	Weight						
	Reps						
	Weight						
	Reps						
	Weight						
	Reps						
	Weight						
	Reps						
	Weight						

Cardio

Exercise	Calories	Distance	Time

Water Intake ___________

Cooldown ___________

Feeling ☆ ☆ ☆ ☆ ☆

Notes

Today's Goal _______________ Ⓜ Ⓣ Ⓦ Ⓣ Ⓕ ● ●

Muscle Group Focus _______________   Weight _______   Date/Time _______

Stretch ◯   Warm-Up _______________________________

Strength Training

Exercise		Set 1	Set 2	Set 3	Set 4	Set 5	Set 6
	Reps						
	Weight						
	Reps						
	Weight						
	Reps						
	Weight						
	Reps						
	Weight						
	Reps						
	Weight						
	Reps						
	Weight						
	Reps						
	Weight						
	Reps						
	Weight						
	Reps						
	Weight						
	Reps						
	Weight						

Cardio

Exercise	Calories	Distance	Time

Water Intake _______________

Cooldown _______________

Feeling ☆ ☆ ☆ ☆ ☆

Notes

Today's Goal ______________ Ⓜ Ⓣ Ⓦ Ⓣ Ⓕ ⬤S ⬤S

Muscle Group Focus ______________   Weight ________   Date/Time __________

Stretch ◯   Warm-Up ________________________________

Strength Training

Exercise		Set 1	Set 2	Set 3	Set 4	Set 5	Set 6
	Reps						
	Weight						
	Reps						
	Weight						
	Reps						
	Weight						
	Reps						
	Weight						
	Reps						
	Weight						
	Reps						
	Weight						
	Reps						
	Weight						
	Reps						
	Weight						
	Reps						
	Weight						

Cardio

Exercise	Calories	Distance	Time

Water Intake ________________

Cooldown ________________

Feeling ☆ ☆ ☆ ☆ ☆

Notes

Today's Goal _______________ Ⓜ Ⓣ Ⓦ Ⓣ Ⓕ ⬤S ⬤S

Muscle Group Focus _______________ Weight _______ Date/Time _______

Stretch ◯   Warm-Up _______________________________

Strength Training

Exercise		Set 1	Set 2	Set 3	Set 4	Set 5	Set 6
	Reps						
	Weight						
	Reps						
	Weight						
	Reps						
	Weight						
	Reps						
	Weight						
	Reps						
	Weight						
	Reps						
	Weight						
	Reps						
	Weight						
	Reps						
	Weight						
	Reps						
	Weight						

Cardio

Exercise	Calories	Distance	Time

Water Intake _______________

Cooldown _______________

Feeling ☆ ☆ ☆ ☆ ☆

Notes

Today's Goal   __________________ Ⓜ Ⓣ Ⓦ Ⓣ Ⓕ ⚫S ⚫S

Muscle Group Focus ________________ Weight ________ Date/Time __________

Stretch ◯   Warm-Up ______________________________________

Strength Training

Exercise		Set 1	Set 2	Set 3	Set 4	Set 5	Set 6
	Reps						
	Weight						
	Reps						
	Weight						
	Reps						
	Weight						
	Reps						
	Weight						
	Reps						
	Weight						
	Reps						
	Weight						
	Reps						
	Weight						
	Reps						
	Weight						
	Reps						
	Weight						
	Reps						
	Weight						

Cardio

Exercise	Calories	Distance	Time

Water Intake __________________

Cooldown __________________

Feeling ☆ ☆ ☆ ☆ ☆

Notes

Today's Goal ____________ (M) (T) (W) (T) (F) (S) (S)

Muscle Group Focus ____________   Weight ________   Date/Time ____________

Stretch ◯   Warm-Up ________________________________

Strength Training

Exercise		Set 1	Set 2	Set 3	Set 4	Set 5	Set 6
	Reps						
	Weight						
	Reps						
	Weight						
	Reps						
	Weight						
	Reps						
	Weight						
	Reps						
	Weight						
	Reps						
	Weight						
	Reps						
	Weight						
	Reps						
	Weight						
	Reps						
	Weight						
	Reps						
	Weight						

Cardio

Exercise	Calories	Distance	Time

Water Intake ____________

Cooldown ____________

Feeling ☆ ☆ ☆ ☆ ☆

Notes

Today's Goal   _____________   (M) (T) (W) (T) (F) (S) (S)

Muscle Group Focus _____________   Weight _______   Date/Time _________

Stretch ◯   Warm-Up _______________________________

Strength Training

Exercise		Set 1	Set 2	Set 3	Set 4	Set 5	Set 6
	Reps						
	Weight						
	Reps						
	Weight						
	Reps						
	Weight						
	Reps						
	Weight						
	Reps						
	Weight						
	Reps						
	Weight						
	Reps						
	Weight						
	Reps						
	Weight						
	Reps						
	Weight						
	Reps						
	Weight						

Cardio

Exercise	Calories	Distance	Time

Water Intake _________________

Cooldown _________________

Feeling ☆ ☆ ☆ ☆ ☆

Notes

Today's Goal _______________ Ⓜ Ⓣ Ⓦ Ⓣ Ⓕ ⬤S ⬤S

Muscle Group Focus _______________ Weight _______ Date/Time _______________

Stretch ◯   Warm-Up _______________

Strength Training

Exercise		Set 1	Set 2	Set 3	Set 4	Set 5	Set 6
	Reps						
	Weight						
	Reps						
	Weight						
	Reps						
	Weight						
	Reps						
	Weight						
	Reps						
	Weight						
	Reps						
	Weight						
	Reps						
	Weight						
	Reps						
	Weight						
	Reps						
	Weight						
	Reps						
	Weight						

Cardio

Exercise	Calories	Distance	Time

Water Intake _______________

Cooldown _______________

Feeling ☆ ☆ ☆ ☆ ☆

Notes

Today's Goal ______________   Ⓜ Ⓣ Ⓦ Ⓣ Ⓕ ● ●

Muscle Group Focus ______________   Weight ________   Date/Time __________

Stretch ◯   Warm-Up ________________________________

Strength Training

Exercise		Set 1	Set 2	Set 3	Set 4	Set 5	Set 6
	Reps						
	Weight						
	Reps						
	Weight						
	Reps						
	Weight						
	Reps						
	Weight						
	Reps						
	Weight						
	Reps						
	Weight						
	Reps						
	Weight						
	Reps						
	Weight						

Cardio

Exercise	Calories	Distance	Time

Water Intake __________________

Cooldown __________________

Feeling ☆ ☆ ☆ ☆ ☆

Notes

Today's Goal __________________ (M) (T) (W) (T) (F) (S) (S)

Muscle Group Focus __________________   Weight _______   Date/Time __________

Stretch ◯   Warm-Up __________________________________

Strength Training

Exercise		Set 1	Set 2	Set 3	Set 4	Set 5	Set 6
	Reps						
	Weight						
	Reps						
	Weight						
	Reps						
	Weight						
	Reps						
	Weight						
	Reps						
	Weight						
	Reps						
	Weight						
	Reps						
	Weight						
	Reps						
	Weight						
	Reps						
	Weight						
	Reps						
	Weight						

Cardio

Exercise	Calories	Distance	Time

Water Intake __________________

Cooldown __________________

Feeling ☆ ☆ ☆ ☆ ☆

Notes

Today's Goal ____________________   Ⓜ Ⓣ Ⓦ Ⓣ Ⓕ ⬤S ⬤S

Muscle Group Focus ________________   Weight ________   Date/Time __________

Stretch ◯   Warm-Up ____

Strength Training

Exercise		Set 1	Set 2	Set 3	Set 4	Set 5	Set 6
	Reps						
	Weight						
	Reps						
	Weight						
	Reps						
	Weight						
	Reps						
	Weight						
	Reps						
	Weight						
	Reps						
	Weight						
	Reps						
	Weight						
	Reps						
	Weight						
	Reps						
	Weight						

Cardio

Exercise	Calories	Distance	Time

Water Intake ________________

Cooldown ________________

Feeling ☆ ☆ ☆ ☆ ☆

Notes

Today's Goal ____________   (M) (T) (W) (T) (F) (S) (S)

Muscle Group Focus ____________   Weight ________   Date/Time ___________

Stretch ◯   Warm-Up ________________________________

Strength Training

Exercise		Set 1	Set 2	Set 3	Set 4	Set 5	Set 6
	Reps						
	Weight						
	Reps						
	Weight						
	Reps						
	Weight						
	Reps						
	Weight						
	Reps						
	Weight						
	Reps						
	Weight						
	Reps						
	Weight						
	Reps						
	Weight						
	Reps						
	Weight						
	Reps						
	Weight						

Cardio

Exercise	Calories	Distance	Time

Water Intake ___________________

Cooldown ___________________

Feeling ☆ ☆ ☆ ☆ ☆

Notes

Today's Goal _______________   Ⓜ Ⓣ Ⓦ Ⓣ Ⓕ ⬤S ⬤S

Muscle Group Focus _______________   Weight _______   Date/Time _______

Stretch ◯   Warm-Up ____

Strength Training

Exercise		Set 1	Set 2	Set 3	Set 4	Set 5	Set 6
	Reps						
	Weight						
	Reps						
	Weight						
	Reps						
	Weight						
	Reps						
	Weight						
	Reps						
	Weight						
	Reps						
	Weight						
	Reps						
	Weight						
	Reps						
	Weight						
	Reps						
	Weight						

Cardio

Exercise	Calories	Distance	Time

Water Intake _________________________

Cooldown _________________________

Feeling ☆ ☆ ☆ ☆ ☆

Notes

Today's Goal ___________________ (M) (T) (W) (T) (F) (S) (S)

Muscle Group Focus ______________ Weight ________ Date/Time __________

Stretch ◯   Warm-Up ____

Strength Training

Exercise		Set 1	Set 2	Set 3	Set 4	Set 5	Set 6
	Reps						
	Weight						
	Reps						
	Weight						
	Reps						
	Weight						
	Reps						
	Weight						
	Reps						
	Weight						
	Reps						
	Weight						
	Reps						
	Weight						
	Reps						
	Weight						
	Reps						
	Weight						
	Reps						
	Weight						

Cardio

Exercise	Calories	Distance	Time

Water Intake _________________

Cooldown _________________

Feeling ☆ ☆ ☆ ☆ ☆

Notes

Today's Goal ____________________ Ⓜ Ⓣ Ⓦ Ⓣ Ⓕ ⚫ ⚫

Muscle Group Focus ______________ Weight ________ Date/Time __________

Stretch ◯ Warm-Up ____

Strength Training

Exercise		Set 1	Set 2	Set 3	Set 4	Set 5	Set 6
	Reps						
	Weight						
	Reps						
	Weight						
	Reps						
	Weight						
	Reps						
	Weight						
	Reps						
	Weight						
	Reps						
	Weight						
	Reps						
	Weight						
	Reps						
	Weight						
	Reps						
	Weight						
	Reps						
	Weight						

Cardio

Exercise	Calories	Distance	Time

Water Intake ____________________

Cooldown ____________________

Feeling ☆ ☆ ☆ ☆ ☆

Notes

Today's Goal _______________ (M) (T) (W) (T) (F) (S) (S)

Muscle Group Focus _______________ Weight ________ Date/Time __________

Stretch ◯ Warm-Up ____

Strength Training

Exercise		Set 1	Set 2	Set 3	Set 4	Set 5	Set 6
	Reps						
	Weight						
	Reps						
	Weight						
	Reps						
	Weight						
	Reps						
	Weight						
	Reps						
	Weight						
	Reps						
	Weight						
	Reps						
	Weight						
	Reps						
	Weight						
	Reps						
	Weight						
	Reps						
	Weight						

Cardio

Exercise	Calories	Distance	Time

Water Intake ________________

Cooldown ________________

Feeling ☆ ☆ ☆ ☆ ☆

Notes

Today's Goal ____________   Ⓜ Ⓣ Ⓦ Ⓣ Ⓕ ⬤S ⬤S

Muscle Group Focus ____________   Weight ______   Date/Time __________

Stretch ◯   Warm-Up ____

Strength Training

Exercise		Set 1	Set 2	Set 3	Set 4	Set 5	Set 6
	Reps						
	Weight						
	Reps						
	Weight						
	Reps						
	Weight						
	Reps						
	Weight						
	Reps						
	Weight						
	Reps						
	Weight						
	Reps						
	Weight						
	Reps						
	Weight						
	Reps						
	Weight						
	Reps						
	Weight						

Cardio

Exercise	Calories	Distance	Time

Water Intake _______________

Cooldown _______________

Feeling ☆ ☆ ☆ ☆ ☆

Notes

Today's Goal _______________ Ⓜ Ⓣ Ⓦ Ⓣ Ⓕ ⬤S ⬤S

Muscle Group Focus _______________   Weight _______   Date/Time _______

Stretch ◯   Warm-Up _________________________________

Strength Training

Exercise		Set 1	Set 2	Set 3	Set 4	Set 5	Set 6
	Reps						
	Weight						
	Reps						
	Weight						
	Reps						
	Weight						
	Reps						
	Weight						
	Reps						
	Weight						
	Reps						
	Weight						
	Reps						
	Weight						
	Reps						
	Weight						
	Reps						
	Weight						
	Reps						
	Weight						

Cardio

Exercise	Calories	Distance	Time

Water Intake _________________

Cooldown _________________

Feeling ☆ ☆ ☆ ☆ ☆

Notes

Today's Goal

Today's Goal _______________ Ⓜ Ⓣ Ⓦ Ⓣ Ⓕ Ⓢ Ⓢ

Muscle Group Focus _______________ Weight _______ Date/Time _______

Stretch ◯ Warm-Up _______________

Strength Training

Exercise		Set 1	Set 2	Set 3	Set 4	Set 5	Set 6
	Reps						
	Weight						
	Reps						
	Weight						
	Reps						
	Weight						
	Reps						
	Weight						
	Reps						
	Weight						
	Reps						
	Weight						
	Reps						
	Weight						
	Reps						
	Weight						
	Reps						
	Weight						
	Reps						
	Weight						

Cardio

Exercise	Calories	Distance	Time

Water Intake _______________

Cooldown _______________

Feeling ☆ ☆ ☆ ☆ ☆

Notes

Today's Goal _______________   Ⓜ Ⓣ Ⓦ Ⓣ Ⓕ ⬤ ⬤

Muscle Group Focus _______________   Weight ________   Date/Time __________

Stretch ◯   Warm-Up _______________________________________

Strength Training

Exercise		Set 1	Set 2	Set 3	Set 4	Set 5	Set 6
	Reps						
	Weight						
	Reps						
	Weight						
	Reps						
	Weight						
	Reps						
	Weight						
	Reps						
	Weight						
	Reps						
	Weight						
	Reps						
	Weight						
	Reps						
	Weight						
	Reps						
	Weight						
	Reps						
	Weight						

Cardio

Exercise	Calories	Distance	Time
_______			
_______			
_______			

Water Intake _______________________

Cooldown _______________________

Feeling ☆ ☆ ☆ ☆ ☆

Notes

Today's Goal ____________ (M) (T) (W) (T) (F) (S) (S)

Muscle Group Focus ____________   Weight ________   Date/Time __________

Stretch ◯   Warm-Up ____________________________________

Strength Training

Exercise		Set 1	Set 2	Set 3	Set 4	Set 5	Set 6
	Reps						
	Weight						
	Reps						
	Weight						
	Reps						
	Weight						
	Reps						
	Weight						
	Reps						
	Weight						
	Reps						
	Weight						
	Reps						
	Weight						
	Reps						
	Weight						
	Reps						
	Weight						
	Reps						
	Weight						

Cardio

Exercise	Calories	Distance	Time

Water Intake ____________________

Cooldown ____________________

Feeling ☆ ☆ ☆ ☆ ☆

Notes

Today's Goal ___________   Ⓜ Ⓣ Ⓦ Ⓣ Ⓕ ● ●

Muscle Group Focus ___________   Weight ______   Date/Time __________

Stretch ◯   Warm-Up ___________________________________

Strength Training

Exercise		Set 1	Set 2	Set 3	Set 4	Set 5	Set 6
	Reps						
	Weight						
	Reps						
	Weight						
	Reps						
	Weight						
	Reps						
	Weight						
	Reps						
	Weight						
	Reps						
	Weight						
	Reps						
	Weight						
	Reps						
	Weight						
	Reps						
	Weight						

Cardio

Exercise	Calories	Distance	Time

Water Intake ___________________

Cooldown ___________________

Feeling ☆ ☆ ☆ ☆ ☆

Notes

Today's Goal ______________   Ⓜ Ⓣ Ⓦ Ⓣ Ⓕ Ⓢ Ⓢ

Muscle Group Focus ______________   Weight ______   Date/Time __________

Stretch ◯   Warm-Up ______________________________

Strength Training

Exercise		Set 1	Set 2	Set 3	Set 4	Set 5	Set 6
	Reps						
	Weight						
	Reps						
	Weight						
	Reps						
	Weight						
	Reps						
	Weight						
	Reps						
	Weight						
	Reps						
	Weight						
	Reps						
	Weight						
	Reps						
	Weight						
	Reps						
	Weight						
	Reps						
	Weight						

Cardio

Exercise	Calories	Distance	Time

Water Intake ______________

Cooldown ______________

Feeling ☆ ☆ ☆ ☆ ☆

Notes

Today's Goal

M T W T F **S** **S**

Muscle Group Focus ___________ Weight ________ Date/Time ________

Stretch ○   Warm-Up ___________

Strength Training

Exercise		Set 1	Set 2	Set 3	Set 4	Set 5	Set 6
	Reps						
	Weight						
	Reps						
	Weight						
	Reps						
	Weight						
	Reps						
	Weight						
	Reps						
	Weight						
	Reps						
	Weight						
	Reps						
	Weight						
	Reps						
	Weight						
	Reps						
	Weight						

Cardio

Exercise	Calories	Distance	Time

Water Intake ___________

Cooldown ___________

Feeling ☆ ☆ ☆ ☆ ☆

Notes